# BEYOND
# REFLECTION

## Bridging Mind and Heart

Anne Bhanu Chopra

Beyond Reflection
Copyright @ 2018 by Anne Bhanu Chopra

First Edition, 2018
Cover Art Direction: Abacho Publishing
Photo Credits: Abacho Publishing

Printed and bound in Canada

Published and distributed by:

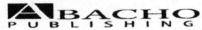

Abacho Publishing
Vancouver, BC

Canadian Cataloguing in Publication Data
Chopra, Anne Bhanu, date.
    Beyond Reflection: Bridging Mind and Heart

ISBN 978-09685694-1-2 (paperback)

1. Conduct of Life--Philosophy   I. Title.
BD431.C4855 2016
128    C2015-905372-2

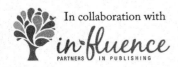 In collaboration with

This book is dedicated to you, my beloved father.

A man of few words, devoted to his principles of clarity, discipline, persistence, loyalty, love, family and forgiveness.

In the last two years of his life, he was challenged by a number of silent strokes. During this time, I had the privilege to share his truths with him each day until his parting. In the most difficult time, he exemplified grace. He continued to fight to live, even while surrendering to the will of nature.

I honor and praise him. He and his teachings remain alive in every cell of my being and this book.

ᥴ~ᥩ

In honor of Dad:

Yesterday I was clever, so I wanted to change the world. Today I am wise, so I am changing myself.

Seek the wisdom that will untie your knot. Seek the path that demands your whole being.

Let yourself be silently drawn by the stronger pull of what you really love.

The wound is the place where the Light enters you.

— Rumi

# Author's Note:

The poet in me evoked, the pen, my instrument challenged to capture the beauty and the complexity of our primal human experience. The pieces reveal the tension between "what is" and "what we wish it to be," the catalyst of the undercurrents and forces of our emotional and physical lives.

My hope is that these pages are a safe place for the readers to reflect, where they find new perspectives of viewing their lives, from both lenses of mind and heart. – **A.B. Chopra**

We read to know that we are not alone. – **C.S. Lewis**

The individual is the picture and the artist.
He is the artist of his personality. – **Alfred Adler**

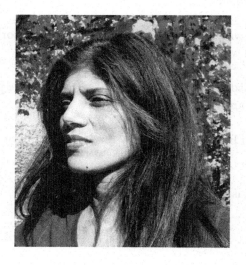

# Praise for:

**Beyond Reflection,** *Bridging Mind and Heart*

This book is a poignant and playful, but ultimately a challenging look at how and why we discover our lives. Both meditative and propulsive, she weaves themes of truth, growth, relationships and love into vignettes that pose questions that are central to navigating human existence.

The pieces crackle with the analytic energy of the trained mind and always in the service of a just heart. Her poetic sensibility provides a lyrical rhythm to philosophic questions that demand intellectual rigour to advance them into the clear light of day. Meaning and understanding are revealed with the gentle grace of words to walk with, wide-eyed and never dogmatic.

Chopra's work intrigues, springing poetry out of the corporate legal boardroom. She gives us a practical companion, a friend to travel with, exercising the mind and nurturing the heart on a journey to personal revelation and wisdom.
**Brian Ball,** *Bookstore Manager, Capilano University, Past President, Campus Stores Canada*

Chopra's writing pulses with life's lyrics. Her astute reflections ripple and riff, like the sun and moon on water, while providing clarity and depth that enlighten the reader.
**Joan Macbeth,** *Screenwriter; Co-writer and Executive Producer of the award-winning documentary, My Shanghai*

Having known and worked alongside Anne Chopra for many years, I have always admired her intelligence and caring nature. Her ability to tap into the universal creative to question and explore the many thoughts that spin through our shared experience, and commit that to writing, is an invitation. In Beyond Reflection, Chopra dedicates her writing to her father making her poem

"Father's Word" particularly poignant, as she pays tribute to his positive and enduring influence on her life. The author's disciplined, curious and gentle mind is abundantly evident as she takes on some of life's toughest issues, and prompts the reader to ask the same questions of themselves. Reflection has many meanings and includes meditative thought but also suggests a reflected image. What do we each see as we gaze into the pond or hold up the mirror? Sometimes it's comforting; sometimes it's harsh; sometimes it's kind; sometimes it's devastating. That is why the quest is bold, and Chopra's writing opens up doors of deeper understanding of life and our place in it. Anne Chopra has accomplished this inspiration as she has grown, changed and sent out a clarion call for us to join her in the exploration of self.
**Hon. Kerry-Lynne D. Findlay,** *QC, J.D., Senior Counsel, Mediator, Speaker, Former Minister of National Revenue*

Anne's writing takes us to universal truths through a passionate, insightful, profound and heartfelt path. She offers us a sense of belonging and connectedness, seamlessly bridging the distance from heart to mind. She soulfully transports us through life's challenges. We want to travel on this journey as her companion. Her writing encourages us to feel, reflect and grow through her words.
**Teal Maedel,** *Registered Psychologist and Past President of the North American Society of Adlerian Psychology, Psychologist for the Correctional Service of Canada*

Chopra's works are authentically raw and beautifully honest. She courageously bears her soul, showing us it's safe for us to look honestly at our own.
**Ashli Komaryk,** *B.A., MBA, Communications Consultant & Certified Trainer (Komaryk Communications)*

Anne has the fine gift of inviting us to consider, with new perspectives, the universal conditions of existence. She describes the dilemmas, contradictions and paradoxes of life in ways that invigorate our energy of curiosity and creativity. She opens the heart to remember and accept what is and to welcome what can be. Anne's powerful use of metaphoric language connects the realities of the wounded soul with spiritful possibilities of life-enriching experiences. With her own life force present in her message, Anne moves us to what we cognitively and intuitively know we need to bring to our doing and being.

**Gloria McArter,** *PhD Registered Clinical Counsellor, Past Director-Workplace Centre for Spiritual/Ethical Development*

Chopra's second book delights, as it is written with the same creativity and sensitivity of her first book. It is an excellent guide for the individual and for a practitioner wanting to unpack the challenges faced by their clients. Her spare prose provides a compass, both moral and compassionate, to those navigating the complexities of an examined life. Anne has deftly presented a broad range of ideas, at times with a light touch, and, when required, with a piercing directness. Her poetic voice will resonate along with the very human wisdom of her perspective.

**Brenlee Carrington Trepel,** *Lawyer, Mediator, Law Society of Manitoba, former Equity Ombudsperson. Free-lance book reviewer, The Winnipeg Free Press since 1998*

Chopra's new book meditates on our existence, to help us live an examined life. She provides unique insights, bridging the gap between the mind and the heart, which propels the reader toward internal freedom. A modern Krishnamurti in the making!

**Dr. Henry M. Codjoe,** *Researcher, Professor-International / Intercultural Education, Director of Institutional Research, Planning and Assessment, Dalton State College*

The pieces in Chopra's second book reminds us of the Ayurvedic approach of aligning with the infinite organizing power of nature - embodied by the Law of Least Effort - rather than struggling to force things. Anne guides us to tap into the intuitive Self, which puts us on an effortless, holistic path. Anne's writing reflects to us that actions motivated by love expend the least effort. So, for the secret to moving to a path of ease, read this book and be guided by love.

**Pamela J. Egger,** *Senior Legal Counsel of a global financial institution, podium awarded athlete, student of spiritual healing and yoga.*

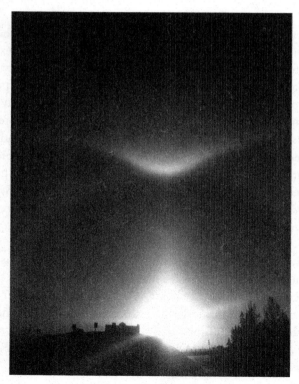

Towards Illumination

# Contents

## Part Eleven:  Love

## Part Twelve:  Voice

## Part Thirteen:  Doing and Being

## Part Fourteen:  Feelings

# Part Fifteen:  Relationships

# Part Sixteen:  Aging

# Part Seventeen:  Reflection

# Foreword

Anne Bhanu Chopra provides the reader with a practical tool to navigate life in the Twenty First Century. The book is a collection of scenarios, 76 in total, each providing a thought-provoking opportunity for an evening of discussion or reflection.

It is intelligent, optimistic, poetic and philosophical. Chopra's compelling and straightforward style is mixed with a subtle sense of humour and is a joy to read. It focuses the reader to mindfully move through modern life.

Anne's writing came to my world when one of my colleagues insisted to keep my copy of her first book, *Beyond the Mirror*. I asked Anne whether she was writing another book that could assist young lawyers struggling with life issues. She shared her latest manuscript *Beyond Reflection*, a poetic compilation for those seeking to understand and optimize life.

Anne has an amazing gift. She has the ability to capture and digest emotions and movements immediately within life moments. In reflecting this back to the reader, *Beyond Reflection* acts as a catalyst, enabling the reader to tap into their personal inner voice of wisdom.

Chopra, the lawyer, has the ability to directly confront the questions inherent in the human condition without fear or hesitation. She creates a safe space, allowing the reader to connect with his or her own vulnerabilities by drawing out the reader's inherent strengths. A sharp intellect, Chopra engages in reflection and deconstruction of life, succeeding in gently moving the reader toward bridging the gap between the mind and heart.

Chopra, the poet, provides Mindsight,©-*weaving together empathy and insight of the human condition.*

As a coach, Chopra reaches out: creating a powerful intimate connection and cultivating an opportunity for self-discovery and change. She leaves the reader with a balanced sense of perspective and tools for understanding the self, others and the world.

Chopra presents a wise, witty and timely book providing the reader with clarity and understanding at a time when there is restlessness, confusion and chaos in the human story.

This book will not collect dust nor can you easily retire it to your shelf after one read. It is a book for your nightstand or coffee table. It is a companion to be shared with your family and friends.

Susan Burak

෴~෴

*Susan Burak, B.A., J. D., M.A., R.C.C., is an Associate Director of Lawyers Assistance Program of British Columbia. In this role she counsels and coaches lawyers and staff with strategic career planning, life transition, anxiety, depression and trauma.*

*Through her education and involvement with a number of international societies and conferences she has both taught and worked with leading experts in the areas of Mindfulness, Neuroscience, Adlerian Psychology, Conflict Resolution and Peace building. Susan is also an adjunct professor at the Adler University, Vancouver Campus and has presented throughout North America, as well as in Ethiopia, Romania, Switzerland and Hungary.*

෴~෴

# Part One

# Open

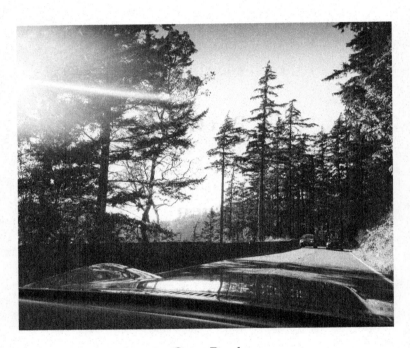

Open Road

# Message of Open

Waves of thoughts,
endeavouring to
message me
to be open.

Pushing
pulling
and propelling me.

I disregard them.
I snub their invite.

They revisit and adamantly say:
    You need us.
    We will assist you.
    Nudging, "be open".

Now I hear the voice of resistance
so persistent:
    please, let me remain, let me be
    I need my comfort
    in my known.

Tension,
of theses voices
conflicting, demanding
delivering and reprimanding.

What do I do?

            ⟷~⟷

## Tension of Voices

The comfort
I attempt to hold on to
remains unfound.

All that exists
is strain
between my existence
and resistance.

Struggle of being open,
louder voices
insisting, fighting
to be heard.

Nothing I can do…
Nothing I can hold on to.

Voices emphatic
eager to take control
make a stand
insist I be open.

Can I be?

## Guiding Messages

Stepping upon life's journey
mind now open...
prepared to listen, to grow
to understand and find meaning
for what is and what is not.

Now exposed to a
multiplicity of philosophies,
messaging their truths:
    no rhyme, no reason,
    happenstance
    random;

    a master plan
    set destiny
    preordained;

    no coincidences
    no accident
    the universe speaks;

    you control
    you are responsible
    author of your life;

    it's all about faith, belief,
    a higher source
    the Provider.

So open, but now so uncertain.

C8~80

## Choosing the Message

We are,
actively or passively
choosing a philosophy.

Choice is ours,
our freedom to choose
our responsibility
holding influence over our lives.

The choice
directs our effort
governs our peace
determines our comfort.

Choosing…
How are we choosing?

C3~80

# Part Two

# Choice

## Book and Story

Choice
in attitude
in the now
in the moment.

What is the story
we are reading
everyday, every night?

Feeding our mind
a story for a time.

Is it a winning one?
Is luck on your side?

Are you leading, a protagonist, or the antagonist
or the victim, or the villain in your story?

Are we choosing a good story for us?
Are we, my friend
aware of this choosing?

The beauty remains...
we have the freedom
to choose
at any time, any moment
a new book, a new role
to be the star
of our new story.

 C3~80

# Mind's Track

Observing some minds
feeling overwhelmed
too responsible
for life's demands
judging the self harshly.

Here to learn,
the path of surrender:
    to let go, to accept what is
    to embrace self-compassion
    to allow for life's command
    to change.

Observing other minds
appearing strong
laying blame outside
never the self
making judgment of life's lot.

Here to learn,
the path of self-accountability:
    to reflect and move from fear
    to be responsible
    to take action
    to change.

What track are you on?  Do you surrender or act?

03~80

## Left Brain Running Wild

I am educated
my learned friend.

Trained to foresee,
schooled against risks.

I understand
the creative mind
can remain
here,
in the now,
what it knows
is enough.

Yes, it can.
It can withstand fear
vulnerability and uncertainty
better than I.

I said I am prepared
trained to foresee
to ask:
    what if ?
    how come?

Now you say, do not ask.
Now you say, just be.
Now you say, what is, just is.

Show me
my learned friend
how to take this mind
to the Now.

What stakes,
what courage it takes
to open the self to judgment—
"you should have known".

I ask, schooling the left-brain
is it safeguarding or depriving us?

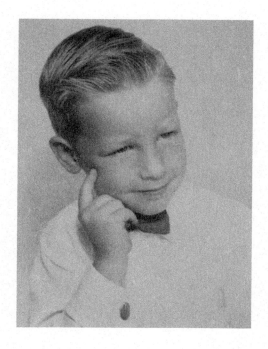

I ask?

## Amplifying Negativity

I see the left-brain attempting
to place us in risk-free boxes.

Fearing the unproven,
amplifying negativity.

Stealing our courage to take risks
losing the growth that comes
with possible failure.

രു~ഇ

# Left Brain Brief

Let us be mindful of the left-brain's expertise, to:

    a) prepare legal briefs;
    b) provide sound judgment; and
    c) safeguard us.

Notwithstanding its qualifications indicated above in paragraph (a), (b) and (c), it should be noted that it activates without authority and is prepared to hijack our life's briefs without our informed consent.

の〜め

## Endings and Worry

Our vision cannot arrive
to the endings that the universe can derive.

Imagination fails us.
Rehearsals of what will be
leave us ill prepared.

Life will ask us
to face
countless unique
and unpredictable endings.
Lives, loves, friendships,
jobs.

Fear does not help.
Worry does not guarantee
success of the rehearsed
we live to fear.

Our dedicated worrying
to a mastered ending
is it preparing us?

ଔ~ଐ

# Part Three

# Gaps

## The Gap

Seeing it.
Feeling it.
Knowing it.

Trusting the existence of it.

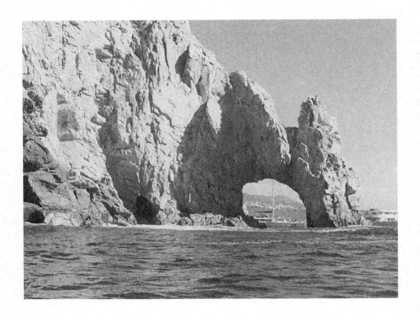

# Gaps

Between words and action.

Between agreement and divergence.

Between beliefs and reality.

Between hearing and understanding.

Identifying the gap
feeling the gap
acting on the gap.

Recognize it.
Know its truth
it exists.

It shall persist
so, do not resist.

03~80

## The Why of the Gap

The gap is here
its existence is known
the reason unknown.

Its plain existence sufficient,
the why not as significant.

 C3~8D

## Pursuing the Why

What is, is.

No apparent reason nor rhyme.
It is what it is.

No need to make time
to pursue
the why.

Take action.
Remove the gap.

I ask, why?

 og~go

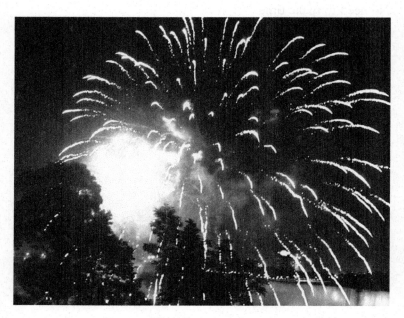

New Beginnings

# Part Four

# Change

# Change at the Table

Old enough,
am I?

To see and know
change is confronted
consistently, carefully
in all spheres.

Change peeks in
gently knocks
seeking permission
to be my guest.

I do not see it
nor hear it
when it knocks
I block it.

I find ways to resist
while it insists!

Undaunted,
change remains determined
to secure my attention.

It breaks my door,
now entering
without manners
without invitation.

Choice is gone
change is here
confronting, pushing me
for a seat at my table.

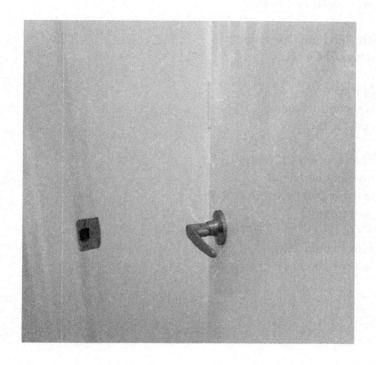

Change Entering

# My Habit, My Friend

To decide to change.

To risk losing you
my suffering
my long-standing habit.

To you, I am devoted
my loyal friend.

Is it true
you comfort me,
console me?

That you, my suffering,
my familiar friend
give me greater comfort than
my struggle?

How would I live
in your absence?

CB~8D

## The Shift

As humans
seeking security
in the known,
wallowing in our habits
at ease, in the realm of the recognized.

We can
make the shift
if we have the hunger.

Create distance,
see our emotions
our reactions,
quash the habitual.

Break free
from this long standing friend
though
she may fight to stop us.

ᐧ❦ᐧ

# Hunger Activated

Some say, change is possible.
Others say
one's past foretells
their future.

I say, it is the hunger
that must be triggered.

Having a hunger
an ache, a longing
a pang
growing so ever strong.

To activate
to trigger
the life of change.

When the "what is"
is insufferable
the hunger emerges.

ଓ~ଟ

# Approaching Change

Modern life
challenges us
slowly, but eventually
commands us to change.

A long life
demands more change.

Sooner or later
it approaches
hits us
while we have endeavoured
to hold on to the "what is."

No fixed blue print
in life
to hold on to.

Holding on
to the "what is"
not an option.

०३~৪०

## Befriending Change

Flexibility, adaptation
openness, resilience
all a part of a wise person's
expanding tool box.

Grasp change
as an instrument of growth
a life force
to thrive
than merely survive.

Prepare to invite
change
knowing its pain
ready to uncover
discover the gains.

I suppose,
those
who embrace change
do indeed have a noble friend.

# Part Five

# Senses

## Sense of Senses

Eyes
blurry,
they cannot see.

Ears
busy,
they cannot hear.

Bones
exhausted,
they cannot move.

I am here
no sense of
eyes, ears and bones.

The state of being.
The state of not.

No sense of being.
No reflection of my being.
No one here.

My friend, help me find
my senses...
my path.

CR~ED

# Clean Lenses

Attachment
to the past
restricting
limiting possibilities
diminishing options.

Limited vision
limited focus
no telescope.

Ample opportunities
for those
who gently
but ever so often
attend to
wash their lenses.

Clean lenses
permit the mind
the eyes
the body
to detach from the past
and attach to the now.

Clean lenses.
Present focused.
Limitless possibilities.
Move forward.

C='~'&)

# Eye to I

Witnessing eyes.

You are the eyes
the lenses
the heart
to capture my I.

Your lenses give me
understanding
definition
reflection.

You bring me to me.
Who I am.
Who I can be.

Your eyes bring me to my I.

CB~&O

# Part Six

# Labels

## Defined

Labels, classifications
all so clean
all so tidy.

Restricting
limiting.

Leaving no space
for fluidity
and the nudity
of the
human in us.

Labels fail
to accept space for the unique.
They define, confine
the spirit
the unexpressed.

CB~BO

# Trapped by the Label

Reader desires
seeks self growth
purchasing books of self-reflection
one after another
creating an impressive library.

Others captivated
by their library
noting the volume of knowledge
presume a reflective soul
presume all has been read.

The books have been opened;
little has been understood.

Constricted, overwhelmed
lost in the labyrinth
frustrated reader
reads,
turns a page
completes one chapter.

Books are quick
to speak to the reader.
Foisting labels, absent consent
trapping the reader.

Remaining chapters
left unread.

೦ಽ~৪৩

## Undefined

Those undefined
remain
fixed and confident
in the known self.

Left alone
to be, to be human
to feel, to reflect
to grow at will
without prescription, book knowledge
or definition.

C3~80

## Examining Labels

*Marked*

Reader is marked
defined clearly by the label
their individuality lost
and labeler's success found.

The labeler
describes and prescribes.
Leaving the reader discouraged
with little room for hope
for prospect for change
or growth.

*Not Marked*

Other readers labeled, but not marked.
A baseline, clarity and value offered.
Purposeful label
help us understand,
express empathy and consideration
for the labeled.

The label is only used for an opening
to find hope, appreciation
for the unique.
Now, opportunities remain
for those labeled
and those labeling.

Within the defined
an individual rests
mindfully
in the awareness
of the undefined.

Unearthing, discovering, expanding
not defining, constricting and limiting.
Enhancing the possibilities
for the labeled and labeler.

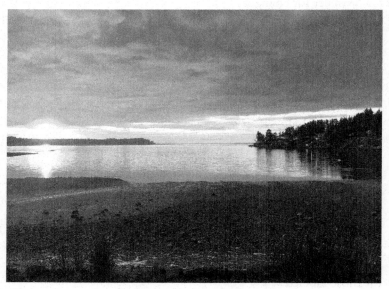

Unearthing Possibilities

# Part Seven

# Discovery

# New Line

Midlife arrives.
Authors, media, and friends
determine authenticity
as the new and better guiding line.

The work is done
student molded
the authentic voice of the child
beaten down…
nowhere to be found.

Counselors step in
ready to assist
to enlist self awareness
to find the lost voice, of truth
our authenticity.

CB~80

# Captive Audience

So shrewd the self-help publisher
focused to create
a captive audience.

Now purchasing a multitude of books.
Reading one after another
to examine
to reflect
to deflect.

This genre of self-help
arming the reader
with knowledge
full of terms
definitions, analysis.

Stripping the reader
of their known
their confidence.
Awakening them to their shadow
the unknown, the masked.

Are we:
    taking these tools to accept the self?
    moving away with book knowledge
    more solid
    more able
    more confident?
    more resourceful, flexible
    leading a contented life?
    finding what we sought?

Not caught in a trap
of self-doubt
fixed to new terms, new knowledge?

Using new-found language
to make presumptions, conclusions
defining and labeling others
based on the latest authority?

Do I have your attention, my captive audience?
Do I?

ᚲᚱ~ᛞᛟ

# Untapped

Untapped, untouched, just being.

Simply, neglected, but free.
Not inundated; absent these messages:
*You need to change.*
*You need to improve.*
*Work on the relationship.*

The untapped
unscathed
walking confident
remaining still
standing tall.

The self-excluded audience
continues to be
the strong
not feeling wrong.

Able to achieve love
as the power resides in them.

Is it so?

CB~80

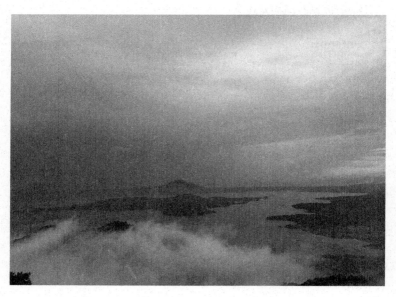

Unbound

# Part Eight

# Freedom

# The Me of Me

Young and fine
full of me.
Slowly
lessons and rules
restricting the me.

Obedience takes hold
compliance with norms
the me of me
chipped away.
I am losing me.

I had my passion
my me,
readily reachable
accessible to all.

Now
the me of me
hidden
deep
buried.

Presentable
pleasing
wrapped package.
Essence forgotten.

෬~෩

## Distractions of the Me

I'm here and
distracted by you.

Much time
being what
you need me to be.

Much time
working on
being
the one I think
you want
me to be.

Gazing in this mirror,
I see her:
 your daughter
 your sister
 your wife
 your lawyer.

I do not readily
see my me.

When I secure my me
my me is here to stay
near, close
sheltered.
Free.

CB~ಞ

# My Child's Me

I see my child,
her me dripping,
readily accessible
to all who meet her.

Her me is everywhere
exposed
in her soul
in speech
her dress
her movements.

She is unrestricted
free, passionate
expressing her me.

I heard her lately
whispering
she is not permitted to say
me words.

She now hears
the cannot, the no words.

You cannot say silly words.
You cannot wear jewelry in school.
You cannot polish your nails.

Small rules, big rules, bigger rules
pleasing parents, teachers
and lovers.

I am praying her me
remains her me
for her and me.

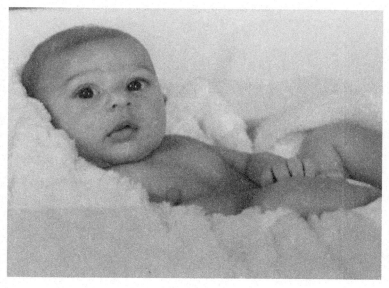

My Me

# Beginner's Mind

Don't lose
the instinctive me
the energy of free
that beginner's mind.

Desire to know.
Desire to grow.

The self regard.
The self to guard.

C8~80

# Part Nine

# Migration

# Migration without Instruction

*The Individual*

Born in a family.
Founded on a land.
Embedded in culture.

Lens for:
What one feels.
What one knows.
What one sees.

*The Dream begins*

The desire for better.
Freedom and wealth.
The hope of more…

*The Passport*

Entering a world
of dissolving boundaries.
where poverty strikes
in words and connection
in meeting expectations.

Walking with limited words on hand.

Timidly peering around:
    new land
    new people
    attempting to understand

the meaning
which words fail to explain.

No one aware of:
    What is not said
    What they do not understand.

Suitcase
of beliefs, culture, family mores and more…

Blindly part taking in this new world.
No guide, no instructions for those
arriving and those inhabiting:
    Words exchanged.
    Nuances missed.
    Culture dismissed.

Language betrays.
Context lost in translation.

What is happening?
Where am I?
Who is this person?
Who is that person?
Why such confusion?

Harsh lessons.
Realizations.
Feeling imperfect in this new world.

*Citizen*

Pause.
Acknowledge ambiguity, confusion, and discomfort.
Unpack suitcase.

Take stock.
what to keep in
what to not?

Discover
    the commonality
    the human being
    the heart
    more than words.

Home at last...
I belong.

 og~&o

# Part Ten

# Connection

## The Nothing and the Everything

With you
the nothing is full of
everything.

With others
the everything gives me
nothing.

෴

## Seconds and Hours

A friendship
where hours of talk feel like
seconds.

With another
seconds in conversation
feel like hours.
And thoughts swarm
to distraction…

ෙ~෧

## Connection and Disconnection

A friendship
where their whole presence fills the room
with the unspoken…
words and comfort.

With another
the silence
chokes me
with its weight.

## Intimacy and Distance

A friendship
where one's ways are delicate nuances
generating
warmth and intimacy.

With another
each habit brings annoyance
creating
distance and doubt.

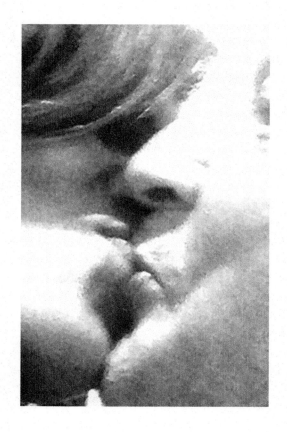

Love's Touch

# Part Eleven

# Love

## The Performer

*Act I:  Drama*

Mastered,
artful performances
moving stage to stage
bearing nothing...
holding fear.

Heart after heart
conquered and trapped
love's imposter has
played the part.

No tears, no regret
proceeding yet
to another stage
another performance
engaging a new heart
a new start.

*Act II:  Audience*

Mystified by the performance
considered as profound
discovering, simply romance.

Giving all.
Believing all.
Risking all.

Failing to see
what is
what is not.

Lights are on
reflection sets in
revealing
what was portrayed:
    the known
    the studied
    the learned
    no more, no less
    no heart.

Disconnection.
Misdirection.
Endless,
going nowhere…

*Act III: Denouement*

Clever, willful
endeavouring art.
Love's imposter
took a heart.

CB~Єⴲ

## Power of it

You control me.
You question me.

I blindly follow
you move me
you move near me
and from me.

You hold me hostage
to your power
to uncertainty.

What are you?

CB~ED

# Elusive Love

Quick moving
whirling and dancing!

Innate essence.
Innate rhythm.

Cannot follow it.
Cannot control it.
Cannot grab it.

Where is it?

Another imposter?

C&~&O

# Love not the Fix

Acts of kindness
sporadically displayed.

You are:
    a cushion of understanding
    a comfort
    a care.

He takes
shares nothing
but his sadness, losses and hurt.

You are not the cause of his resounding fear.
You are just the ear.

Run, they say run
run quick.

There is no space
for you in his place.

You are ready for love
but, they are in need of a fix.

Hurt by timing
and his space.

No connection
misdirection.

Should you stay?
Give it time?
Give understanding?

Should you be the fix
when you belong to love?

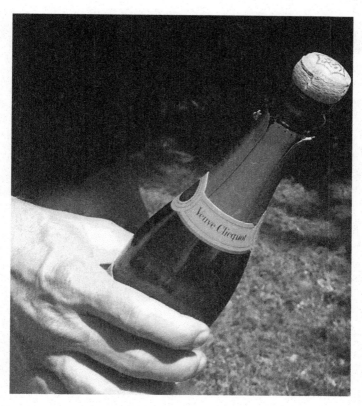

Love or the Fix?

## Sense and Fear

Can sense it.
Cannot make sense of it.

We know we long for it.
We are strong for it.
Slaving so long for it.

It appears,
we lust for it
dominating
we have fear
and no trust for it.

It disappears,
alone again
insecure in its absence
yearning for its return.

ᨄ~ᨃ

# No Definition

I have no definition of it.
I have not found it.

I have a picture of it.
I continue searching for it.
I have moments of it.

So I follow it.
Was it here?

08~80

## Love's Will

Love seeks truth
breeds generosity
extends understanding
lives beyond.

A broken smile
an injured heart
love remains relentless.

It has courage.
It rises.
It takes charge
removes losses
without fail.

It moves to share.
It works to heal.
It has its will.

It shall shelter.
It shall protect
whosoever it finds.

CB~ED

# Part Twelve

# Voice

## Voice in the Gaps

Whose voice?
What voice
 is filling the gaps:
    in conversation
    in communication
    with yourself
    with others?

Your voice?
Her voice?
His voice?

Is it the voice of fear or that of love?

03~80

## Voice of Love

Love seeks to unearth
a forgiving explanation
a generous interpretation
laced with empathy, understanding.

Never concealing
what it is.
Never pretending
to be
more than it is.

Love's voice
fills gaps
with courage and strength,
seeking means of connection.

When love catches itself
feeling insecure
afraid, vulnerable
it is willing to reveal its truth
in courage to itself and others.

C3~80

# Fear's Voice

The voice of fear
dances, appears like love
but ultimately
reveals its self.

Fear hides
safeguarding
with assorted masks.

The pure voice of fear
holds shame at its core.

Never able to appear
without its shield of confidence
its loyal guise.

Dancing in with coolness
pretending to be love.

Fear's thoughts are born
with measuring, withholding
detachment
all at its core.

Hedging
never at ease.
Fearing, concealing
the pain, the truth.
Making those near
uncertain, and unsure.

CB~ED

## Anatomy of Fear

Looking closer
using lenses
deconstructing.

We see that fear
in its essence
in its elements
has an absence, a scarcity
a lack of belief.

Fear's constitution is perfection.
Freezing growth
leaving no space for:
    self-acceptance
    acknowledgement of truths
    pain, insecurity, failures
all aspects of the human condition.

ଓ~ଚ

## Moving Voice

A decision made
conscious, unconscious
to secure a mask
one of survival.

Raised in a world of fear
not hearing the word of love.

Now exposed
we have heard love's voice
we can move
from fear to there.

Our choice,
we can learn
to move
to remove
our mask of fear
encasing shame or endless blame.

Embrace a new found voice
moving forward
with courage.

ℭ~ℬ

# Part Thirteen

# Doing and Being

## Doing and Being

### Task 1

They are on the go.
They are doing.

They are the doers.

### Task 2

They move.
They compartmentalize.

Make tasks out of nothing.
Line up projects where none exist.

### Task 3

They don't question.
They memorize.
They are in the business of doing.

No time to reflect.
Time to deflect.

### Task 4

They don't worry.
They do more.

They don't personalize.
Time to rationalize.

**Task 5**

Moving forward.
Clock ticking.
Time defined.

New game.
New score.
One more point.
It's a win.

Is it?

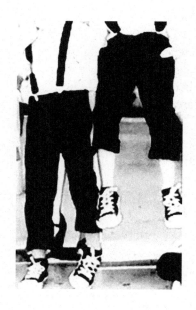

The Shoes of Doing

# Choke Me Here in the Shallow End

Memorize, compete, challenge—find the answer.

Win, work and spar-- by showing the other up.

Who said it?

When was it written?

Who sang it?

What was the score?

What was the date?

You tell me this is important.
You tell me you are smart.

I say
Google has the answers.

Can we be still?
Still use our minds
for reflection?

Can we?

෴~෴

# Educated Self

I listen to her
she listens to me.

Our stories start differently
yet we arrive
at the very same space.

She has her education
independence
health and wealth.

We share
we compare
we have much in common
we seek the same goal.

We work to secure the imagined.
A goal so simple, yet
it finds ways to elude us.

With our strength
our conviction
we work, we endeavour
we do not surrender.

She finds means
to improve us.
I undertake her journey
of educating us.

At the end of our self governed PhD
the books have succeeded.

They have accomplished
their task
they have won.
We now have a questioning self
and lost our confident one.

Our task
our goal
remains elusive.

But, I understand
we have grown.
A new language known
new terms
new labels
and endless definitions.

Undeniably educated...
Are we brighter?

☙~❧

# Part Fourteen

# Feelings

## Confined Feelings

Feelings,
life forces
relegated to unreachable
tight, defined, confined places.

Appearing alive
breathing air
but not life.

Restricted.
Do not enter. Stop!
Signage properly situated
holding feelings
to their inaccessible place.

ᛣ~ᛠ

# Doing

Respect for feelings
the strength
the truth
the expression.

Not accustomed to this
in our world.

We live where tangible sought
intangible discarded.

What are we doing instead?

May I humbly say
we are doing "doing" well.

03~80

## Doing and Drinking

Many tired of the doing
permitted to exit
the doing by drinking.

Under the guise of doing a drink,
more able
to move
to travel
to reach
the concealed place
where our feelings lie.

ભ~જ

## Containers

Self contained,
emotions under control
measured
fully discerned.

Show just enough.
Give just enough.
Be just enough.

Am I mistaken?
Here I stand
without my suit
yet ruled by the realm of business.

No, this is the new guiding light
approaching
now encroaching upon us.

Pressing us to contain feelings.
Everywhere, anywhere …

I am.
I am contained.
I am the container.

०३~८०

# Uncontained

Permitted
we are
to remove
the mask.

Are we not?

I appreciate the drink
provides permission
to remove our mask
in the social realm.

The drink,
a renowned justification
to divulge
the clandestine
our emotions
our truths, our content
our story.

Of course,
one can also take a lie
on the counselor's couch
no justification required
no drink in hand
uninhibited disclosure
resistance gone
uncontained.
Permission granted.

෯~෧

## Feeling

The art of feeling.
The permission to feel.
The place to feel.

To feel in our bodies.
To feel in our bones.
To feel in our hearts.

Honour feelings
their rightful place
not hidden nor
forbidden.

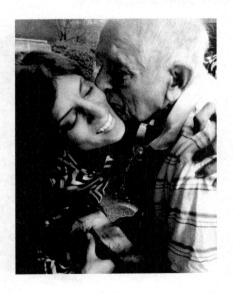

Love's Honesty

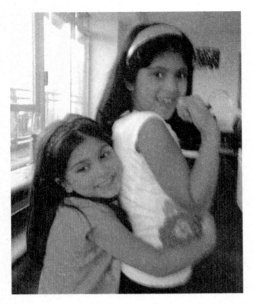

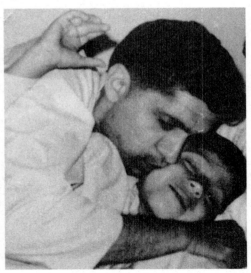

Bonds

# Part Fifteen

# Relationships

# Wrong Company Strong Will

Come confident, bring your will.

Find a companion
commit to a road
principles in hand
each of their own.

Holding strong
walking a road
faithful to its principles
not permitting the exit...

On this road
one grows stronger
another grows weaker.

Time passes blindly.

Time to reassess
the hold of this road
the hold of the principles.

My friend,
your principles, your will
are they honoured
on your chosen road?

# Freedom of Without

To walk at your own pace.

To find your humour.
To find your taste.

To uncover the self
rediscover
you are enough.

Give freedom to be
to take your freedom
to be without
no verdict
no judgment
let us be.

ଓଃ~ଽଠ

## Strength's Secret

I have a secret, a form.
I have something
I truly guard.

Allows me to be
allows me to smile
to cry
to be free.

Every time I connect
it generates, regenerates
memoirs and more.

Resulting in a belonging
a strength, a bonding.
Restoring the soul
generating joy.

Nothing measured
no roles
no prescriptions
accepts my errors
shields me from hurt.

This gift, I do covet.

In truth and trust
in pain and forgiveness
furnishing strength to my form.

Many have it.
Some want it.
Many seek it.
Some run from it.

Priceless,
under appreciated
under celebrated.

Family
with its pain and love
survives
thrives
and remains.

Family is in blood
in friendship
in community.

In the moment
of giving, taking
and making the time:
    to connect
    to understand
    to forgive, to flow
we create our family.

Remember me always
your family, your strength
in your form.

ᘓ~ᘔ

## Father's Word

A father,
a man of his word
giving one's word is gold.

Disciplined,
in mind and action
open heart.

Do not say something
you do not intend,
say less.

Be mindful when speaking,
if you say it,
you have promised
you must honour it.

There is no trying,
there is only doing.

This, my Indian father
fair and tall
raised by the English
resides in me.

Time after time
the mind hears
a father's words.

Their messaging
their guidance
their love.

Growing and desiring
to find my own way.

But, they insist
on revisiting me.

In my mind
my father's words
reside.
Golden words
hold me steady.

Able to trust
able to love
absent fear
as he, and his words
are always near.

Father's words
remain alive.

CB~80

## Texture not Logic

Woven for one.
Ready to be
where none would go.

No one understands.
No one comprehends.

All make presumptions,
none satisfy.

Logic fails to explain
why you remain.
Yet, texture rises
claims the connection.

CŞ~ŞꝹ

# The We

The strength of the we
woven with the connection of two me(s).

Time, space and devotion
creating a lasting we.

Able and willing
to work on the weave,
reaping the vigor and verve
of being a we.

Honoring the we
the me holds privilege
of belonging to the we.

ᑕ᙭~᙭ᑐ

## Inescapable We

Hurt by the we.
Unable to see
the need for the we.

Holding tight to the me
allowing no space to weave the we.

Safe,
living in the fear of the we
surviving me.

Inescapable,
to thrive
we must be open
to weave the we.

⊂⊱~⊰⊃

# Part Sixteen

# Aging

## Commanded Beauty

Older, and we know it
but not permitted to show it.

Commanded to conceal
what grace lines reveal.

A forced beauty
is upon us
a new aim of our time.

The fight of aging
instilling fear
short life for wrinkles
no place for grace
middle age shattered.

03~80

# Hijacked Mind

Heart filled youth
beating, in spirit
with life.

Face conscious
older, wiser
displaying a life.

The mind speaks its mind
powerfully
keeping its confidence.

Hijacked,
making demands:
   be disciplined
    secure your youth.

Mind not mine
fear moved in
media messages governing
commanding commitment.

⊂⊱~⊰⊃

## Nature's Mirror

Media
takes hold
exploiting fears
inducing minds
invalidating confidence.

Stealing our compass.
Reliance on nature's law
no longer an option.

Wrinkles, fine lines
expressions
never find their graceful start.

Creams, lotions, botox
assorted procedures
invading and ruling lives.

Nature not permitted
to play its God given role
providing gentle reminders
of time's wisdom.

Mirrors unable
to relay the naked truths.
Beauty now confused.

ಞ~ಲ

## Stolen Grace

So you,
who have bought us
the face of youth
I hear we should have no fear.

Advanced treatments
creams, potions and endless
solutions.

A multitude of choices
no fear.
New questions:
    which one?
    how many?
    how much?

We are relieved from aging
in a new realm of staging.

Now a new concern
as to whether we have done enough
to secure the new face of youth
as grace has been stolen
from our face of aging.

03~80

## Fragile Friend hello, Goodbye Wisdom lines

Now I have you
I am uncertain
insecure as to how
to hold on to you.

Face of youth
my fragile friend
you require constant reassurances
of I having done enough.

My loyal friend, time
displays its friendship
with lines of wisdom.
I apologize.

I have been too eager for my new friend,
remiss with you.
Blindly disregarding you,
your wisdom, and grace
by removing any trace of our friendship.

ભ~♥

## Studying Him

At 82, he is vibrant.
Confident, articulate.
Handsome.
Lean
a professional
suit, tie and polished shoes
aging
no illness
no clues.

Breakfast made to style.
Walking tall to work
helping his clients
with their files.

Illness knocked
a silent stroke
took hold
silenced,
words no more.

Diminished health
Grace holding all.

I look at him
study him.

His hands
his eyes
his movements.

Each action
any sound
all distinct.

Without notice,
much taken
his form forsaken.

He is my dad,
he is my father.

I see your dad,
he is your father.

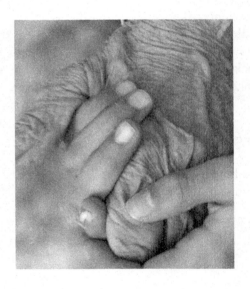

Hands of Generations

# New Form

The stroke brings new form
no speech, no words
we do not converse
in the usual form.

He thinks
revealing his thoughts
speaking with his eyes.

He connects
with those in his life
giving him time
trusting in him
in his soul, in his essence
not in his new form.

For those who see
more than his form
they shall meet
a soulful soul
a gift of light
the presence of grace
with its tender embrace.

ℭ৪~৪ℭ

## Suspended Goodbye

Walking...
Pain resides inside.

Feeling him leaving.

Part of him leaving.
Part of him staying.

Is he leaving?

Everyday
panic strikes.

He then amazes me.
He is stronger.

Using his will
to surrender to what is
he is here,
in no rush to leave
radiating life.

He is not leaving
still breathing.

Resilient, he is striving
more than surviving
in his new form.

He is feeling strong
but for how long?

I can breathe and be
but can I be?

Is he leaving? No one knows.

Suspended parting.
Suspending goodbye.

No haste for him to leave.

Living this privilege, facing him
his existence:
    his pain
    mother's pain
    my pain
    life's pain.

The privilege, the blessing
to live the suspended goodbye.
A universal capacity
to give, to love
while pain takes residence in you.

Pain, I say to you
thank you
for finding me
letting me see you
so I could embrace the blessing
of living the suspended goodbye.

☙~❧

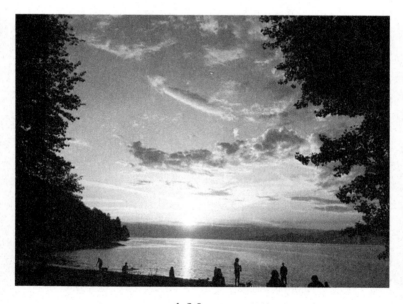

A Moment

# Part Seventeen

# Reflection

## Speaking to Time

We say, stand still to time
when in joy's place.
Hours pass as moments
days pass as hours.

We beg time to pass
when in pain's place.
Minutes pass as days
days pass as months.

Yes, time
it has its own mind
travels
on its own time.

 G~80

# Time Speaks

Now older
time speaks louder
at a racing speed.

Months pass as days.
Years pass as weeks.

I say, have patience with me
I am not the young
eagerly awaiting for you to pass.

I have had a change of heart.
I beg you to go slow...

Time
when did you tell me
you would run
at such a pace
and with such haste?

಄~ೞ

# Acknowledgement

I give a special thanks to my editors, Brian, and Joan. Embracing this project from beginning to end. They patiently worked with me from the early versions to this stage and providing encouragement, gentle confrontations and valuable feedback.

I have an abundance of gratitude for my friend, colleague Susan Burak for her hard work, dedication and unfailing enthusiasm.

I'm very thankful to Sherry Siu and Cynthia Chan for her generosity of time and talent in formatting this book.

For hours of conversations, thought and review that went to the heart of the book: Suneela, Ashli, Pamela, Joan, Andrew and Brian.

A sincere thanks to all those friends and colleagues for offering their support and encouragement: Alma, Brenlee, David, Ron, Tim, John, Hector, Savita, and Paul.

Boundless appreciation to: my brother and sister, Mani and Suneela; my nephews, Aarun and Nishal, my nieces Angelia and Pryianka, who acted as my special project director, with wisdom beyond her years.

And lastly, I give my love and thanks to my partner, Randy, my dearest Mother and to the memory of my Father for their endless love and support.

I did not write this book alone, it is with great pleasure and privilege that I share my writings with you.

C8~80

## About the Author

Anne Bhanu Chopra, B.Comm., M.I.R. (Queen's) J.D., is a corporate lawyer, public company director, lecturer, coach & law society ombudsperson. In 1999 she published her first book, *Beyond the Mirror- Seeing Ourselves As We Are.*

Alison Azer, in the University of Alberta Business Magazine 2004, described this book as *"examining human existence through an intimate voice of reflection and advice"*.

For 18 years Chopra was the ombudsperson for the Law Society of British Columbia, providing conflict resolution, education, coaching and training to individuals and firms. She is committed to bringing the analytical framework of the corporate world into the complex human dynamics prevalent in the realm of coaching and the workplace. Anne lives in Vancouver, British Columbia.

## Also Written by Anne Chopra:

*Beyond the Mirror, Seeing Ourselves As We Are*, 1999.

# Contact Author

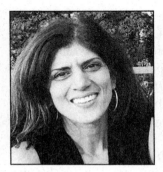

Email: achopra1@novuscom.net
Phone: (604) 812-2344
Website: www.annechopra.com

*My hope is that this book becomes your companion. Enriches you by providing you the space to hear and find your inner voice of wisdom.*